Blood Sugar Tracker

~weekly set up to track daily readings
~ includes images to color for your enjoyment

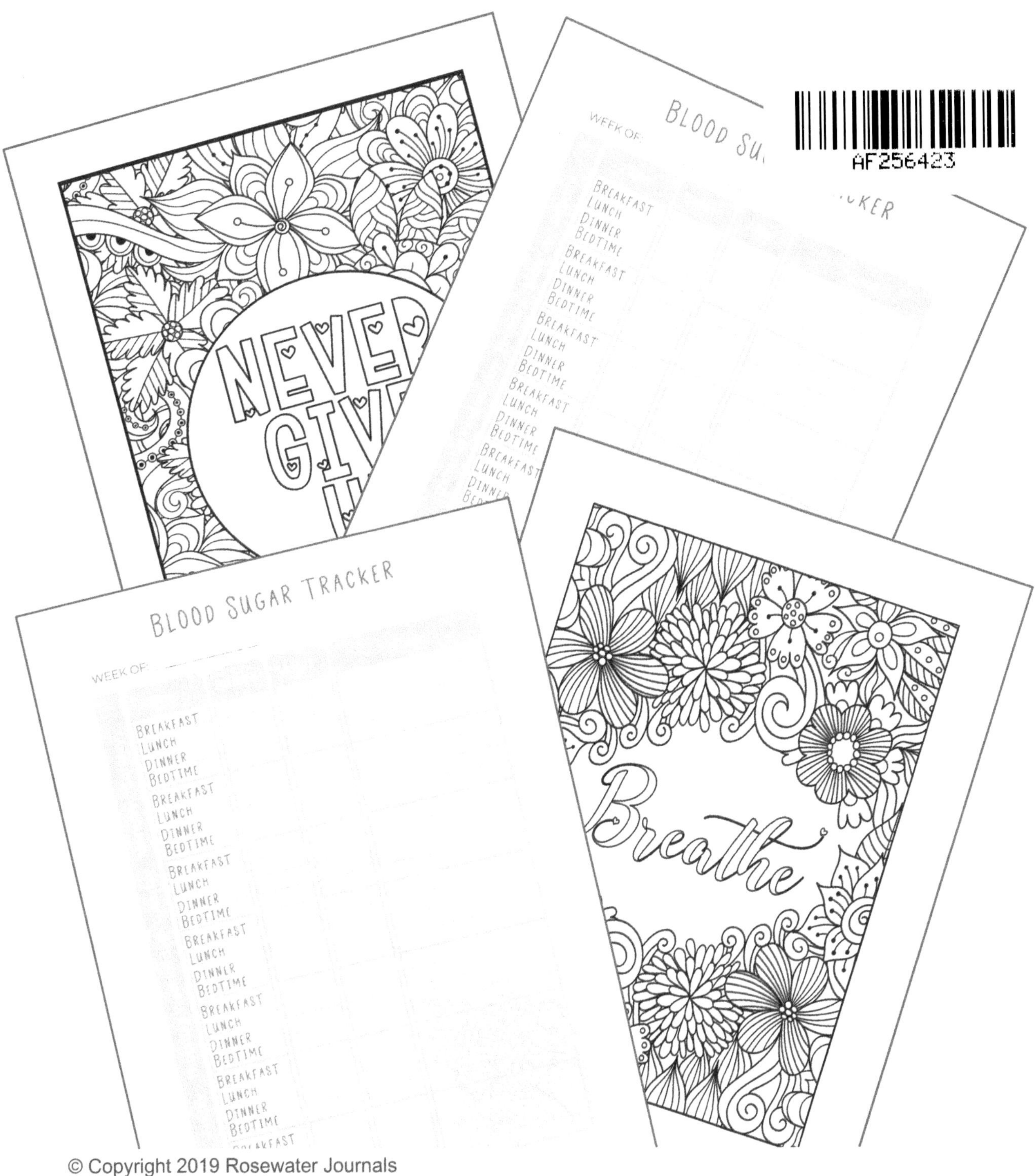

© Copyright 2019 Rosewater Journals

All rights reserved.

This book or any portion thereof may not be reproduced or used in any manner whatsoever without the express written permission of the publisher except for the use of brief quotations in a book review.

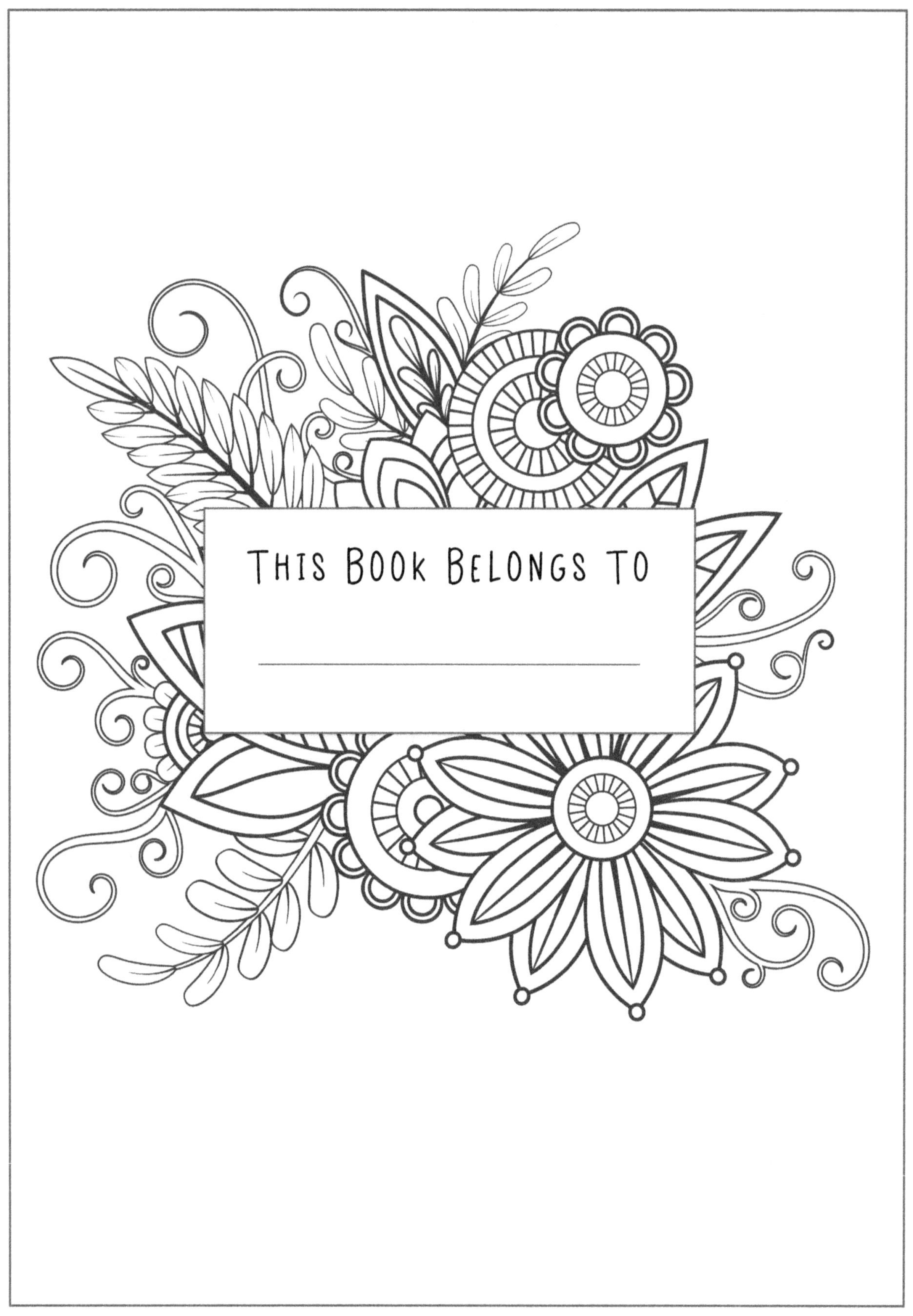

THIS BOOK BELONGS TO

Blood Sugar Tracker

WEEK OF: _______________________

	Before	After	Notes
Breakfast			
Lunch			
Dinner			
Bedtime			
Breakfast			
Lunch			
Dinner			
Bedtime			
Breakfast			
Lunch			
Dinner			
Bedtime			
Breakfast			
Lunch			
Dinner			
Bedtime			
Breakfast			
Lunch			
Dinner			
Bedtime			
Breakfast			
Lunch			
Dinner			
Bedtime			
Breakfast			
Lunch			
Dinner			
Bedtime			

Blood Sugar Tracker

WEEK OF: _________________

	Time	Before	After	Notes
Sunday	Breakfast Lunch Dinner Bedtime			
Monday	Breakfast Lunch Dinner Bedtime			
Tuesday	Breakfast Lunch Dinner Bedtime			
Wednesday	Breakfast Lunch Dinner Bedtime			
Thursday	Breakfast Lunch Dinner Bedtime			
Friday	Breakfast Lunch Dinner Bedtime			
Saturday	Breakfast Lunch Dinner Bedtime			

Blood Sugar Tracker

WEEK OF: ___________________

Time	Before	After	Notes
Breakfast			
Lunch			
Dinner			
Bedtime			
Breakfast			
Lunch			
Dinner			
Bedtime			
Breakfast			
Lunch			
Dinner			
Bedtime			
Breakfast			
Lunch			
Dinner			
Bedtime			
Breakfast			
Lunch			
Dinner			
Bedtime			
Breakfast			
Lunch			
Dinner			
Bedtime			
Breakfast			
Lunch			
Dinner			
Bedtime			

Blood Sugar Tracker

WEEK OF: _______________________

	Time	Before	After	Notes
Sunday	Breakfast			
	Lunch			
	Dinner			
	Bedtime			
Monday	Breakfast			
	Lunch			
	Dinner			
	Bedtime			
Tuesday	Breakfast			
	Lunch			
	Dinner			
	Bedtime			
Wednesday	Breakfast			
	Lunch			
	Dinner			
	Bedtime			
Thursday	Breakfast			
	Lunch			
	Dinner			
	Bedtime			
Friday	Breakfast			
	Lunch			
	Dinner			
	Bedtime			
Saturday	Breakfast			
	Lunch			
	Dinner			
	Bedtime			

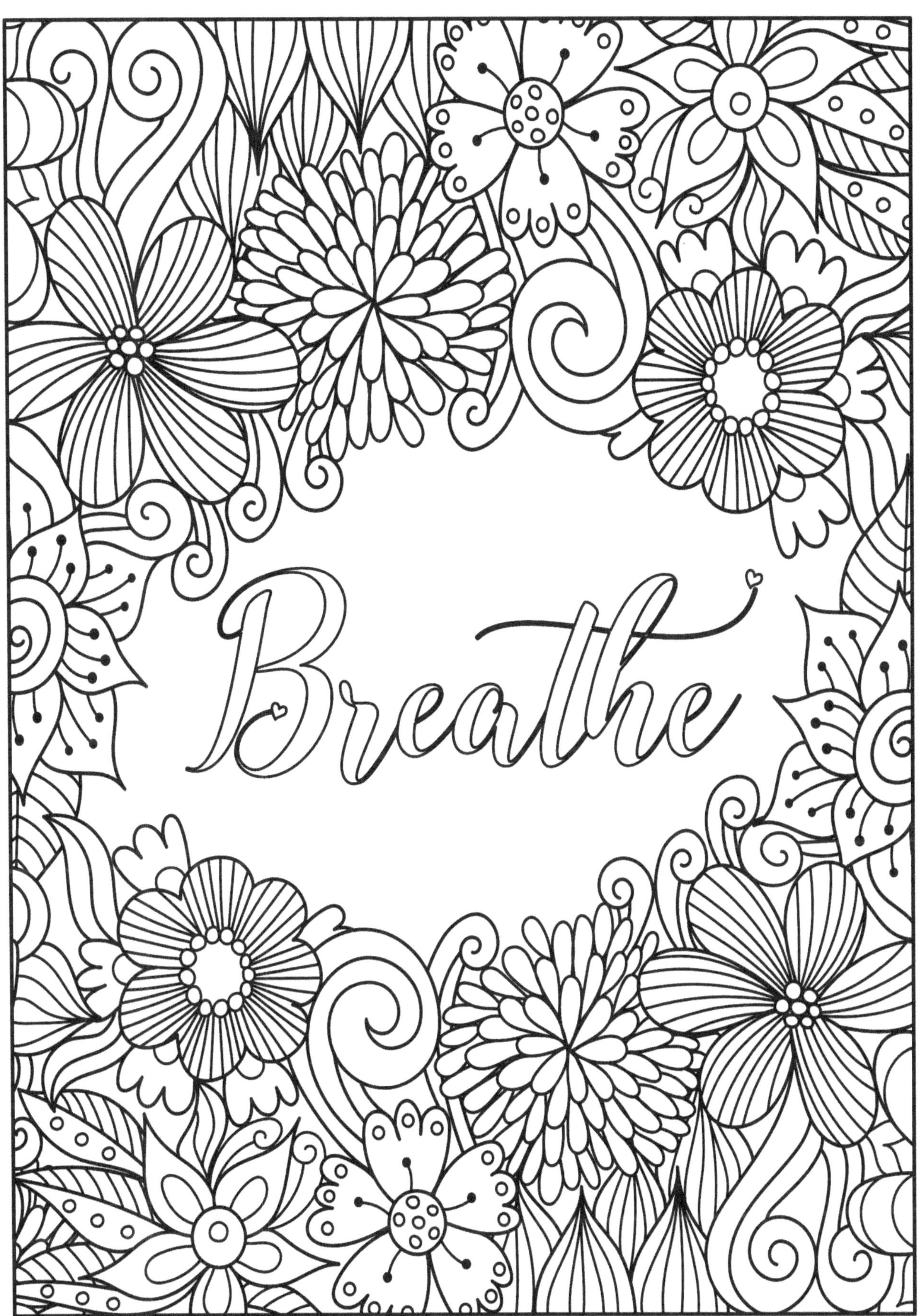
Breathe

Blood Sugar Tracker

WEEK OF: ___________________

Time	Before	After	Notes
Breakfast			
Lunch			
Dinner			
Bedtime			
Breakfast			
Lunch			
Dinner			
Bedtime			
Breakfast			
Lunch			
Dinner			
Bedtime			
Breakfast			
Lunch			
Dinner			
Bedtime			
Breakfast			
Lunch			
Dinner			
Bedtime			
Breakfast			
Lunch			
Dinner			
Bedtime			
Breakfast			
Lunch			
Dinner			
Bedtime			

Blood Sugar Tracker

WEEK OF: _______________

Time	Before	After	Notes
Breakfast			
Lunch			
Dinner			
Bedtime			
Breakfast			
Lunch			
Dinner			
Bedtime			
Breakfast			
Lunch			
Dinner			
Bedtime			
Breakfast			
Lunch			
Dinner			
Bedtime			
Breakfast			
Lunch			
Dinner			
Bedtime			
Breakfast			
Lunch			
Dinner			
Bedtime			
Breakfast			
Lunch			
Dinner			
Bedtime			

BLOOD SUGAR TRACKER

WEEK OF: _______________

	TIME	BEFORE	AFTER	NOTES
	BREAKFAST			
	LUNCH			
	DINNER			
	BEDTIME			
	BREAKFAST			
	LUNCH			
	DINNER			
	BEDTIME			
	BREAKFAST			
	LUNCH			
	DINNER			
	BEDTIME			
	BREAKFAST			
	LUNCH			
	DINNER			
	BEDTIME			
	BREAKFAST			
	LUNCH			
	DINNER			
	BEDTIME			
	BREAKFAST			
	LUNCH			
	DINNER			
	BEDTIME			
	BREAKFAST			
	LUNCH			
	DINNER			
	BEDTIME			

Blood Sugar Tracker

WEEK OF: _______________________

Time	Before	After	Notes
BREAKFAST			
LUNCH			
DINNER			
BEDTIME			
BREAKFAST			
LUNCH			
DINNER			
BEDTIME			
BREAKFAST			
LUNCH			
DINNER			
BEDTIME			
BREAKFAST			
LUNCH			
DINNER			
BEDTIME			
BREAKFAST			
LUNCH			
DINNER			
BEDTIME			
BREAKFAST			
LUNCH			
DINNER			
BEDTIME			
BREAKFAST			
LUNCH			
DINNER			
BEDTIME			

NOTES:

Blood Sugar Tracker

WEEK OF: _______________

Time	Before	After	Notes
Breakfast			
Lunch			
Dinner			
Bedtime			
Breakfast			
Lunch			
Dinner			
Bedtime			
Breakfast			
Lunch			
Dinner			
Bedtime			
Breakfast			
Lunch			
Dinner			
Bedtime			
Breakfast			
Lunch			
Dinner			
Bedtime			
Breakfast			
Lunch			
Dinner			
Bedtime			
Breakfast			
Lunch			
Dinner			
Bedtime			

Blood Sugar Tracker

WEEK OF: ______________________

	Time	Before	After	Notes
Sunday	Breakfast Lunch Dinner Bedtime			
Monday	Breakfast Lunch Dinner Bedtime			
Tuesday	Breakfast Lunch Dinner Bedtime			
Wednesday	Breakfast Lunch Dinner Bedtime			
Thursday	Breakfast Lunch Dinner Bedtime			
Friday	Breakfast Lunch Dinner Bedtime			
Saturday	Breakfast Lunch Dinner Bedtime			

Blood Sugar Tracker

WEEK OF: ___________________

	Time	Before	After	Notes
Sunday	Breakfast			
	Lunch			
	Dinner			
	Bedtime			
Monday	Breakfast			
	Lunch			
	Dinner			
	Bedtime			
Tuesday	Breakfast			
	Lunch			
	Dinner			
	Bedtime			
Wednesday	Breakfast			
	Lunch			
	Dinner			
	Bedtime			
Thursday	Breakfast			
	Lunch			
	Dinner			
	Bedtime			
Friday	Breakfast			
	Lunch			
	Dinner			
	Bedtime			
Saturday	Breakfast			
	Lunch			
	Dinner			
	Bedtime			

BLOOD SUGAR TRACKER

WEEK OF: _______________________

	Time	Before	After	Notes
Sunday	Breakfast			
	Lunch			
	Dinner			
	Bedtime			
Monday	Breakfast			
	Lunch			
	Dinner			
	Bedtime			
Tuesday	Breakfast			
	Lunch			
	Dinner			
	Bedtime			
Wednesday	Breakfast			
	Lunch			
	Dinner			
	Bedtime			
Thursday	Breakfast			
	Lunch			
	Dinner			
	Bedtime			
Friday	Breakfast			
	Lunch			
	Dinner			
	Bedtime			
Saturday	Breakfast			
	Lunch			
	Dinner			
	Bedtime			

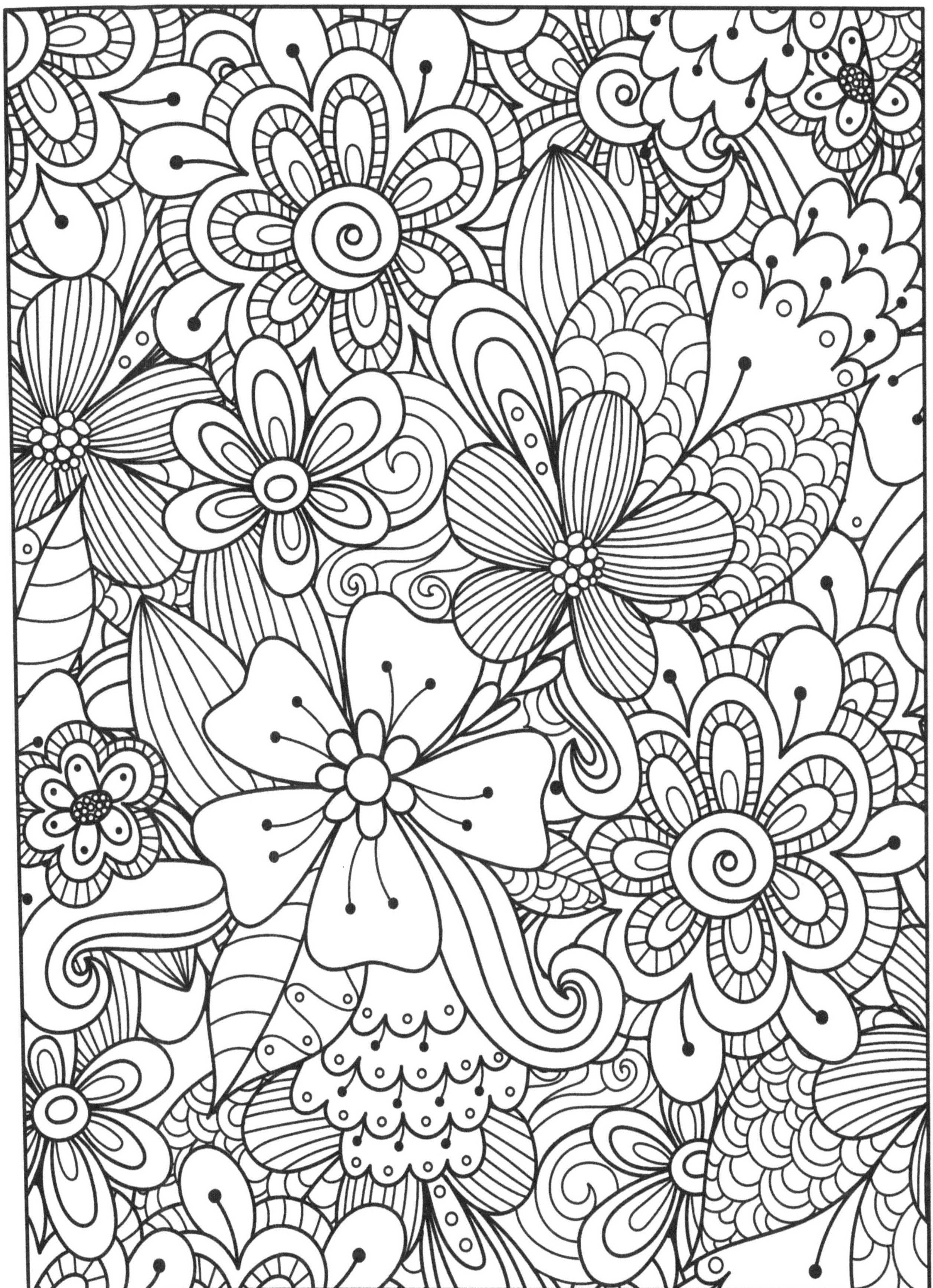

Blood Sugar Tracker

WEEK OF: _______________

	Time	Before	After	Notes
Sunday	Breakfast Lunch Dinner Bedtime			
Monday	Breakfast Lunch Dinner Bedtime			
Tuesday	Breakfast Lunch Dinner Bedtime			
Wednesday	Breakfast Lunch Dinner Bedtime			
Thursday	Breakfast Lunch Dinner Bedtime			
Friday	Breakfast Lunch Dinner Bedtime			
Saturday	Breakfast Lunch Dinner Bedtime			

Blood Sugar Tracker

WEEK OF: _______________________

	Time	Before	After	Notes
Sunday	Breakfast			
	Lunch			
	Dinner			
	Bedtime			
Monday	Breakfast			
	Lunch			
	Dinner			
	Bedtime			
Tuesday	Breakfast			
	Lunch			
	Dinner			
	Bedtime			
Wednesday	Breakfast			
	Lunch			
	Dinner			
	Bedtime			
Thursday	Breakfast			
	Lunch			
	Dinner			
	Bedtime			
Friday	Breakfast			
	Lunch			
	Dinner			
	Bedtime			
Saturday	Breakfast			
	Lunch			
	Dinner			
	Bedtime			

Blood Sugar Tracker

WEEK OF: _______________

	Time	Before	After	Notes
	Breakfast			
	Lunch			
	Dinner			
	Bedtime			
	Breakfast			
	Lunch			
	Dinner			
	Bedtime			
	Breakfast			
	Lunch			
	Dinner			
	Bedtime			
	Breakfast			
	Lunch			
	Dinner			
	Bedtime			
	Breakfast			
	Lunch			
	Dinner			
	Bedtime			
	Breakfast			
	Lunch			
	Dinner			
	Bedtime			
	Breakfast			
	Lunch			
	Dinner			
	Bedtime			

Blood Sugar Tracker

WEEK OF: _______________________

<table>
<tr><td></td><td>Time</td><td>Before</td><td>After</td><td>Notes</td></tr>
<tr><td rowspan="4">Sunday</td><td>Breakfast</td><td></td><td></td><td></td></tr>
<tr><td>Lunch</td><td></td><td></td><td></td></tr>
<tr><td>Dinner</td><td></td><td></td><td></td></tr>
<tr><td>Bedtime</td><td></td><td></td><td></td></tr>
<tr><td rowspan="4">Monday</td><td>Breakfast</td><td></td><td></td><td></td></tr>
<tr><td>Lunch</td><td></td><td></td><td></td></tr>
<tr><td>Dinner</td><td></td><td></td><td></td></tr>
<tr><td>Bedtime</td><td></td><td></td><td></td></tr>
<tr><td rowspan="4">Tuesday</td><td>Breakfast</td><td></td><td></td><td></td></tr>
<tr><td>Lunch</td><td></td><td></td><td></td></tr>
<tr><td>Dinner</td><td></td><td></td><td></td></tr>
<tr><td>Bedtime</td><td></td><td></td><td></td></tr>
<tr><td rowspan="4">Wednesday</td><td>Breakfast</td><td></td><td></td><td></td></tr>
<tr><td>Lunch</td><td></td><td></td><td></td></tr>
<tr><td>Dinner</td><td></td><td></td><td></td></tr>
<tr><td>Bedtime</td><td></td><td></td><td></td></tr>
<tr><td rowspan="4">Thursday</td><td>Breakfast</td><td></td><td></td><td></td></tr>
<tr><td>Lunch</td><td></td><td></td><td></td></tr>
<tr><td>Dinner</td><td></td><td></td><td></td></tr>
<tr><td>Bedtime</td><td></td><td></td><td></td></tr>
<tr><td rowspan="4">Friday</td><td>Breakfast</td><td></td><td></td><td></td></tr>
<tr><td>Lunch</td><td></td><td></td><td></td></tr>
<tr><td>Dinner</td><td></td><td></td><td></td></tr>
<tr><td>Bedtime</td><td></td><td></td><td></td></tr>
<tr><td rowspan="4">Saturday</td><td>Breakfast</td><td></td><td></td><td></td></tr>
<tr><td>Lunch</td><td></td><td></td><td></td></tr>
<tr><td>Dinner</td><td></td><td></td><td></td></tr>
<tr><td>Bedtime</td><td></td><td></td><td></td></tr>
</table>

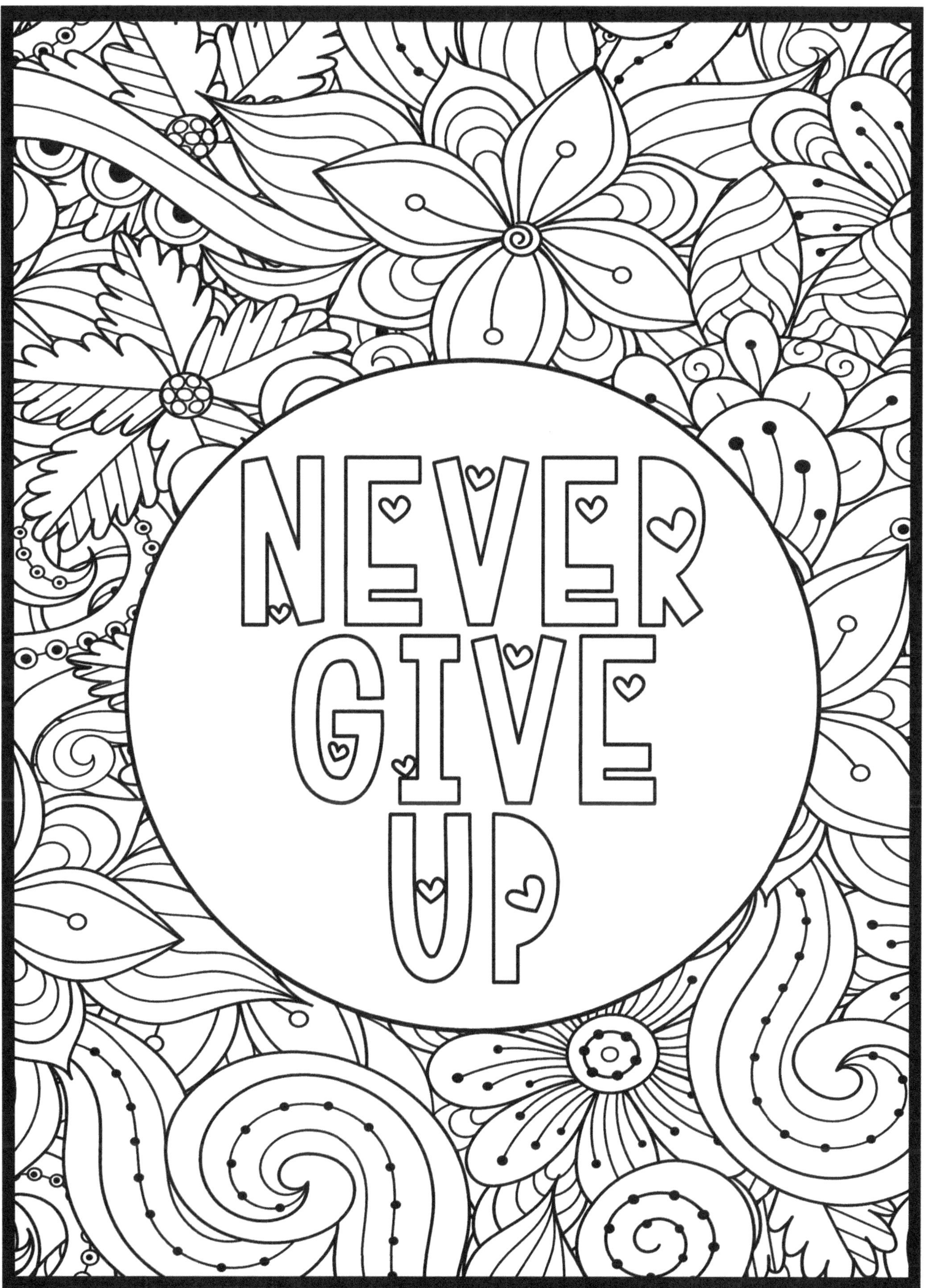

NEVER
GIVE
UP

Blood Sugar Tracker

WEEK OF: _________________

	Time	Before	After	Notes
	Breakfast			
	Lunch			
	Dinner			
	Bedtime			
	Breakfast			
	Lunch			
	Dinner			
	Bedtime			
	Breakfast			
	Lunch			
	Dinner			
	Bedtime			
	Breakfast			
	Lunch			
	Dinner			
	Bedtime			
	Breakfast			
	Lunch			
	Dinner			
	Bedtime			
	Breakfast			
	Lunch			
	Dinner			
	Bedtime			
	Breakfast			
	Lunch			
	Dinner			
	Bedtime			

Blood Sugar Tracker

WEEK OF: _______________________

Time	Before	After	Notes
Breakfast			
Lunch			
Dinner			
Bedtime			
Breakfast			
Lunch			
Dinner			
Bedtime			
Breakfast			
Lunch			
Dinner			
Bedtime			
Breakfast			
Lunch			
Dinner			
Bedtime			
Breakfast			
Lunch			
Dinner			
Bedtime			
Breakfast			
Lunch			
Dinner			
Bedtime			
Breakfast			
Lunch			
Dinner			
Bedtime			

Blood Sugar Tracker

WEEK OF: _____________________

	Time	Before	After	Notes
Sunday	Breakfast			
	Lunch			
	Dinner			
	Bedtime			
Monday	Breakfast			
	Lunch			
	Dinner			
	Bedtime			
Tuesday	Breakfast			
	Lunch			
	Dinner			
	Bedtime			
Wednesday	Breakfast			
	Lunch			
	Dinner			
	Bedtime			
Thursday	Breakfast			
	Lunch			
	Dinner			
	Bedtime			
Friday	Breakfast			
	Lunch			
	Dinner			
	Bedtime			
Saturday	Breakfast			
	Lunch			
	Dinner			
	Bedtime			

Blood Sugar Tracker

WEEK OF: _______________________

Day	Time	Before	After	Notes
Sunday	Breakfast			
	Lunch			
	Dinner			
	Bedtime			
Monday	Breakfast			
	Lunch			
	Dinner			
	Bedtime			
Tuesday	Breakfast			
	Lunch			
	Dinner			
	Bedtime			
Wednesday	Breakfast			
	Lunch			
	Dinner			
	Bedtime			
Thursday	Breakfast			
	Lunch			
	Dinner			
	Bedtime			
Friday	Breakfast			
	Lunch			
	Dinner			
	Bedtime			
Saturday	Breakfast			
	Lunch			
	Dinner			
	Bedtime			

NOTES:

Blood Sugar Tracker

WEEK OF: _______________________

Time	Before	After	Notes
Breakfast			
Lunch			
Dinner			
Bedtime			
Breakfast			
Lunch			
Dinner			
Bedtime			
Breakfast			
Lunch			
Dinner			
Bedtime			
Breakfast			
Lunch			
Dinner			
Bedtime			
Breakfast			
Lunch			
Dinner			
Bedtime			
Breakfast			
Lunch			
Dinner			
Bedtime			
Breakfast			
Lunch			
Dinner			
Bedtime			

Blood Sugar Tracker

WEEK OF: ___________________

	Time	Before	After	Notes
Sunday	Breakfast			
	Lunch			
	Dinner			
	Bedtime			
Monday	Breakfast			
	Lunch			
	Dinner			
	Bedtime			
Tuesday	Breakfast			
	Lunch			
	Dinner			
	Bedtime			
Wednesday	Breakfast			
	Lunch			
	Dinner			
	Bedtime			
Thursday	Breakfast			
	Lunch			
	Dinner			
	Bedtime			
Friday	Breakfast			
	Lunch			
	Dinner			
	Bedtime			
Saturday	Breakfast			
	Lunch			
	Dinner			
	Bedtime			

Blood Sugar Tracker

WEEK OF: ________________________

	Time	Before	After	Notes
	Breakfast Lunch Dinner Bedtime			
	Breakfast Lunch Dinner Bedtime			
	Breakfast Lunch Dinner Bedtime			
	Breakfast Lunch Dinner Bedtime			
	Breakfast Lunch Dinner Bedtime			
	Breakfast Lunch Dinner Bedtime			
	Breakfast Lunch Dinner Bedtime			

BLOOD SUGAR TRACKER

WEEK OF: _______________________

	Time	Before	After	Notes
Sunday	BREAKFAST			
	LUNCH			
	DINNER			
	BEDTIME			
Monday	BREAKFAST			
	LUNCH			
	DINNER			
	BEDTIME			
Tuesday	BREAKFAST			
	LUNCH			
	DINNER			
	BEDTIME			
Wednesday	BREAKFAST			
	LUNCH			
	DINNER			
	BEDTIME			
Thursday	BREAKFAST			
	LUNCH			
	DINNER			
	BEDTIME			
Friday	BREAKFAST			
	LUNCH			
	DINNER			
	BEDTIME			
Saturday	BREAKFAST			
	LUNCH			
	DINNER			
	BEDTIME			

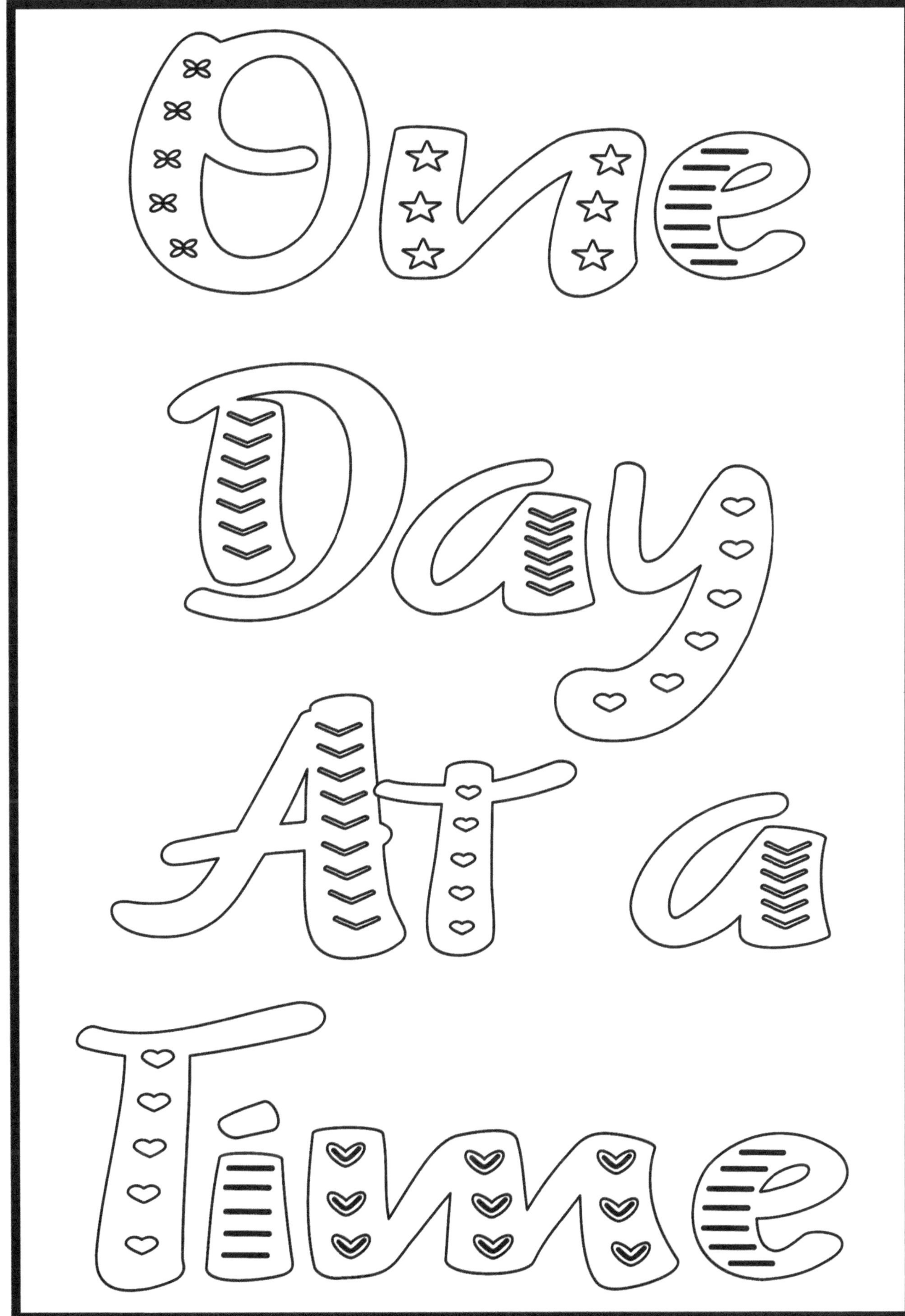

One
Day
At a
Time

Blood Sugar Tracker

WEEK OF: _______________________

Time	Before	After	Notes
Breakfast			
Lunch			
Dinner			
Bedtime			
Breakfast			
Lunch			
Dinner			
Bedtime			
Breakfast			
Lunch			
Dinner			
Bedtime			
Breakfast			
Lunch			
Dinner			
Bedtime			
Breakfast			
Lunch			
Dinner			
Bedtime			
Breakfast			
Lunch			
Dinner			
Bedtime			
Breakfast			
Lunch			
Dinner			
Bedtime			

Blood Sugar Tracker

WEEK OF: _______________

<table>
<tr><td rowspan="28">Saturday Friday Thursday Wednesday Tuesday Monday Sunday</td><td>Time</td><td>Before</td><td>After</td><td>Notes</td></tr>
<tr><td>Breakfast</td><td></td><td></td><td></td></tr>
<tr><td>Lunch</td><td></td><td></td><td></td></tr>
<tr><td>Dinner</td><td></td><td></td><td></td></tr>
<tr><td>Bedtime</td><td></td><td></td><td></td></tr>
<tr><td>Breakfast</td><td></td><td></td><td></td></tr>
<tr><td>Lunch</td><td></td><td></td><td></td></tr>
<tr><td>Dinner</td><td></td><td></td><td></td></tr>
<tr><td>Bedtime</td><td></td><td></td><td></td></tr>
<tr><td>Breakfast</td><td></td><td></td><td></td></tr>
<tr><td>Lunch</td><td></td><td></td><td></td></tr>
<tr><td>Dinner</td><td></td><td></td><td></td></tr>
<tr><td>Bedtime</td><td></td><td></td><td></td></tr>
<tr><td>Breakfast</td><td></td><td></td><td></td></tr>
<tr><td>Lunch</td><td></td><td></td><td></td></tr>
<tr><td>Dinner</td><td></td><td></td><td></td></tr>
<tr><td>Bedtime</td><td></td><td></td><td></td></tr>
<tr><td>Breakfast</td><td></td><td></td><td></td></tr>
<tr><td>Lunch</td><td></td><td></td><td></td></tr>
<tr><td>Dinner</td><td></td><td></td><td></td></tr>
<tr><td>Bedtime</td><td></td><td></td><td></td></tr>
<tr><td>Breakfast</td><td></td><td></td><td></td></tr>
<tr><td>Lunch</td><td></td><td></td><td></td></tr>
<tr><td>Dinner</td><td></td><td></td><td></td></tr>
<tr><td>Bedtime</td><td></td><td></td><td></td></tr>
<tr><td>Breakfast</td><td></td><td></td><td></td></tr>
<tr><td>Lunch</td><td></td><td></td><td></td></tr>
<tr><td>Dinner</td><td></td><td></td><td></td></tr>
<tr><td>Bedtime</td><td></td><td></td><td></td></tr>
</table>

Blood Sugar Tracker

WEEK OF: ________________

Time	Before	After	Notes
Breakfast			
Lunch			
Dinner			
Bedtime			
Breakfast			
Lunch			
Dinner			
Bedtime			
Breakfast			
Lunch			
Dinner			
Bedtime			
Breakfast			
Lunch			
Dinner			
Bedtime			
Breakfast			
Lunch			
Dinner			
Bedtime			
Breakfast			
Lunch			
Dinner			
Bedtime			
Breakfast			
Lunch			
Dinner			
Bedtime			

Blood Sugar Tracker

WEEK OF: _____________________

	Time	Before	After	Notes
Sunday	Breakfast			
	Lunch			
	Dinner			
	Bedtime			
Monday	Breakfast			
	Lunch			
	Dinner			
	Bedtime			
Tuesday	Breakfast			
	Lunch			
	Dinner			
	Bedtime			
Wednesday	Breakfast			
	Lunch			
	Dinner			
	Bedtime			
Thursday	Breakfast			
	Lunch			
	Dinner			
	Bedtime			
Friday	Breakfast			
	Lunch			
	Dinner			
	Bedtime			
Saturday	Breakfast			
	Lunch			
	Dinner			
	Bedtime			

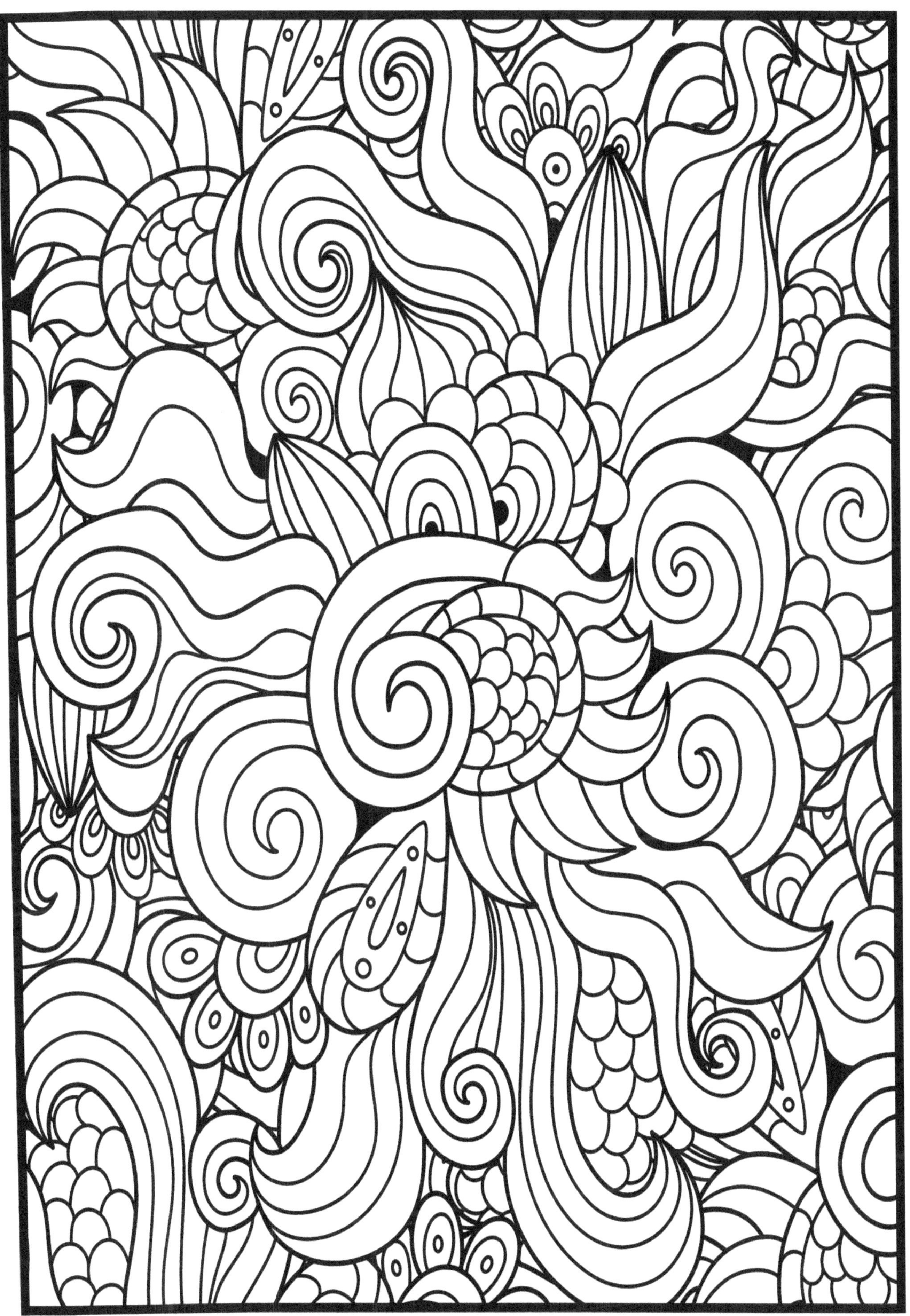

Blood Sugar Tracker

WEEK OF: _______________

Day	Time	Before	After	Notes
Sunday	Breakfast			
	Lunch			
	Dinner			
	Bedtime			
Monday	Breakfast			
	Lunch			
	Dinner			
	Bedtime			
Tuesday	Breakfast			
	Lunch			
	Dinner			
	Bedtime			
Wednesday	Breakfast			
	Lunch			
	Dinner			
	Bedtime			
Thursday	Breakfast			
	Lunch			
	Dinner			
	Bedtime			
Friday	Breakfast			
	Lunch			
	Dinner			
	Bedtime			
Saturday	Breakfast			
	Lunch			
	Dinner			
	Bedtime			

Blood Sugar Tracker

WEEK OF: _________________

	Time	Before	After	Notes
Sunday	Breakfast			
	Lunch			
	Dinner			
	Bedtime			
Monday	Breakfast			
	Lunch			
	Dinner			
	Bedtime			
Tuesday	Breakfast			
	Lunch			
	Dinner			
	Bedtime			
Wednesday	Breakfast			
	Lunch			
	Dinner			
	Bedtime			
Thursday	Breakfast			
	Lunch			
	Dinner			
	Bedtime			
Friday	Breakfast			
	Lunch			
	Dinner			
	Bedtime			
Saturday	Breakfast			
	Lunch			
	Dinner			
	Bedtime			

Blood Sugar Tracker

WEEK OF: ______________________

Time	Before	After	Notes
Breakfast			
Lunch			
Dinner			
Bedtime			
Breakfast			
Lunch			
Dinner			
Bedtime			
Breakfast			
Lunch			
Dinner			
Bedtime			
Breakfast			
Lunch			
Dinner			
Bedtime			
Breakfast			
Lunch			
Dinner			
Bedtime			
Breakfast			
Lunch			
Dinner			
Bedtime			
Breakfast			
Lunch			
Dinner			
Bedtime			

Blood Sugar Tracker

WEEK OF: _______________

Time	Before	After	Notes
Breakfast			
Lunch			
Dinner			
Bedtime			
Breakfast			
Lunch			
Dinner			
Bedtime			
Breakfast			
Lunch			
Dinner			
Bedtime			
Breakfast			
Lunch			
Dinner			
Bedtime			
Breakfast			
Lunch			
Dinner			
Bedtime			
Breakfast			
Lunch			
Dinner			
Bedtime			
Breakfast			
Lunch			
Dinner			
Bedtime			

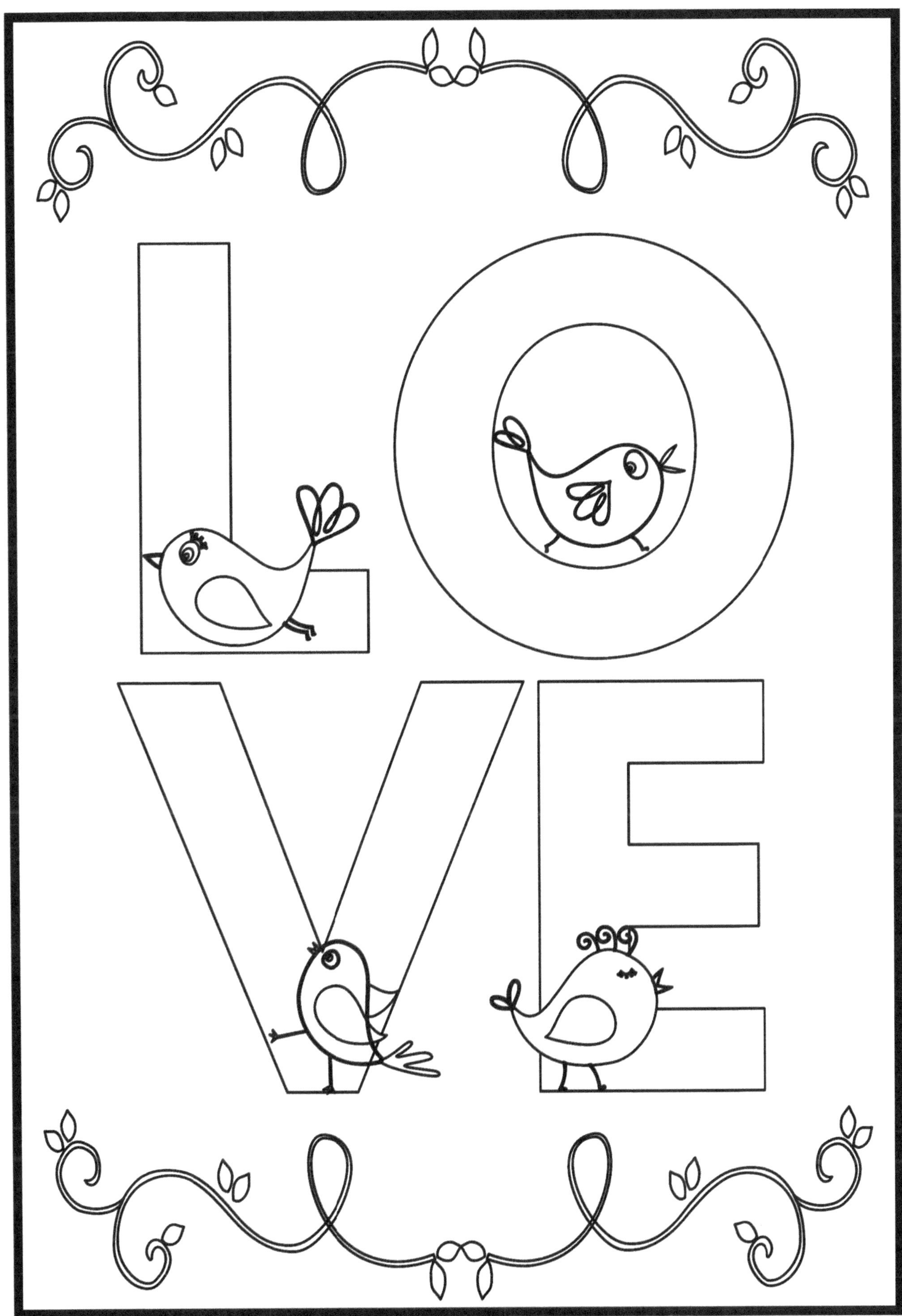

Blood Sugar Tracker

WEEK OF: _______________________

	Time	Before	After	Notes
Sunday	Breakfast Lunch Dinner Bedtime			
Monday	Breakfast Lunch Dinner Bedtime			
Tuesday	Breakfast Lunch Dinner Bedtime			
Wednesday	Breakfast Lunch Dinner Bedtime			
Thursday	Breakfast Lunch Dinner Bedtime			
Friday	Breakfast Lunch Dinner Bedtime			
Saturday	Breakfast Lunch Dinner Bedtime			

Blood Sugar Tracker

WEEK OF: _______________________

	Time	Before	After	Notes
Sunday	Breakfast			
	Lunch			
	Dinner			
	Bedtime			
Monday	Breakfast			
	Lunch			
	Dinner			
	Bedtime			
Tuesday	Breakfast			
	Lunch			
	Dinner			
	Bedtime			
Wednesday	Breakfast			
	Lunch			
	Dinner			
	Bedtime			
Thursday	Breakfast			
	Lunch			
	Dinner			
	Bedtime			
Friday	Breakfast			
	Lunch			
	Dinner			
	Bedtime			
Saturday	Breakfast			
	Lunch			
	Dinner			
	Bedtime			

Blood Sugar Tracker

WEEK OF: _________________

Time	Before	After	Notes
Breakfast			
Lunch			
Dinner			
Bedtime			
Breakfast			
Lunch			
Dinner			
Bedtime			
Breakfast			
Lunch			
Dinner			
Bedtime			
Breakfast			
Lunch			
Dinner			
Bedtime			
Breakfast			
Lunch			
Dinner			
Bedtime			
Breakfast			
Lunch			
Dinner			
Bedtime			
Breakfast			
Lunch			
Dinner			
Bedtime			

Blood Sugar Tracker

WEEK OF: _______________________

	Time	Before	After	Notes
Sunday	Breakfast			
	Lunch			
	Dinner			
	Bedtime			
Monday	Breakfast			
	Lunch			
	Dinner			
	Bedtime			
Tuesday	Breakfast			
	Lunch			
	Dinner			
	Bedtime			
Wednesday	Breakfast			
	Lunch			
	Dinner			
	Bedtime			
Thursday	Breakfast			
	Lunch			
	Dinner			
	Bedtime			
Friday	Breakfast			
	Lunch			
	Dinner			
	Bedtime			
Saturday	Breakfast			
	Lunch			
	Dinner			
	Bedtime			

NOTES:

Blood Sugar Tracker

WEEK OF: _________________

	Time	Before	After	Notes
Sunday	Breakfast			
	Lunch			
	Dinner			
	Bedtime			
Monday	Breakfast			
	Lunch			
	Dinner			
	Bedtime			
Tuesday	Breakfast			
	Lunch			
	Dinner			
	Bedtime			
Wednesday	Breakfast			
	Lunch			
	Dinner			
	Bedtime			
Thursday	Breakfast			
	Lunch			
	Dinner			
	Bedtime			
Friday	Breakfast			
	Lunch			
	Dinner			
	Bedtime			
Saturday	Breakfast			
	Lunch			
	Dinner			
	Bedtime			

Blood Sugar Tracker

WEEK OF: _______________________

Time	Before	After	Notes
Breakfast			
Lunch			
Dinner			
Bedtime			
Breakfast			
Lunch			
Dinner			
Bedtime			
Breakfast			
Lunch			
Dinner			
Bedtime			
Breakfast			
Lunch			
Dinner			
Bedtime			
Breakfast			
Lunch			
Dinner			
Bedtime			
Breakfast			
Lunch			
Dinner			
Bedtime			
Breakfast			
Lunch			
Dinner			
Bedtime			

Blood Sugar Tracker

WEEK OF: ____________________

	Time	Blood	After	Notes
	Breakfast			
	Lunch			
	Dinner			
	Bedtime			
	Breakfast			
	Lunch			
	Dinner			
	Bedtime			
	Breakfast			
	Lunch			
	Dinner			
	Bedtime			
	Breakfast			
	Lunch			
	Dinner			
	Bedtime			
	Breakfast			
	Lunch			
	Dinner			
	Bedtime			
	Breakfast			
	Lunch			
	Dinner			
	Bedtime			
	Breakfast			
	Lunch			
	Dinner			
	Bedtime			

Blood Sugar Tracker

WEEK OF: _______________________

<table>
<tr><td></td><td>Time</td><td>Before</td><td>After</td><td>Notes</td></tr>
<tr><td rowspan="4">Sunday</td><td>Breakfast</td><td></td><td></td><td></td></tr>
<tr><td>Lunch</td><td></td><td></td><td></td></tr>
<tr><td>Dinner</td><td></td><td></td><td></td></tr>
<tr><td>Bedtime</td><td></td><td></td><td></td></tr>
<tr><td rowspan="4">Monday</td><td>Breakfast</td><td></td><td></td><td></td></tr>
<tr><td>Lunch</td><td></td><td></td><td></td></tr>
<tr><td>Dinner</td><td></td><td></td><td></td></tr>
<tr><td>Bedtime</td><td></td><td></td><td></td></tr>
<tr><td rowspan="4">Tuesday</td><td>Breakfast</td><td></td><td></td><td></td></tr>
<tr><td>Lunch</td><td></td><td></td><td></td></tr>
<tr><td>Dinner</td><td></td><td></td><td></td></tr>
<tr><td>Bedtime</td><td></td><td></td><td></td></tr>
<tr><td rowspan="4">Wednesday</td><td>Breakfast</td><td></td><td></td><td></td></tr>
<tr><td>Lunch</td><td></td><td></td><td></td></tr>
<tr><td>Dinner</td><td></td><td></td><td></td></tr>
<tr><td>Bedtime</td><td></td><td></td><td></td></tr>
<tr><td rowspan="4">Thursday</td><td>Breakfast</td><td></td><td></td><td></td></tr>
<tr><td>Lunch</td><td></td><td></td><td></td></tr>
<tr><td>Dinner</td><td></td><td></td><td></td></tr>
<tr><td>Bedtime</td><td></td><td></td><td></td></tr>
<tr><td rowspan="4">Friday</td><td>Breakfast</td><td></td><td></td><td></td></tr>
<tr><td>Lunch</td><td></td><td></td><td></td></tr>
<tr><td>Dinner</td><td></td><td></td><td></td></tr>
<tr><td>Bedtime</td><td></td><td></td><td></td></tr>
<tr><td rowspan="4">Saturday</td><td>Breakfast</td><td></td><td></td><td></td></tr>
<tr><td>Lunch</td><td></td><td></td><td></td></tr>
<tr><td>Dinner</td><td></td><td></td><td></td></tr>
<tr><td>Bedtime</td><td></td><td></td><td></td></tr>
</table>

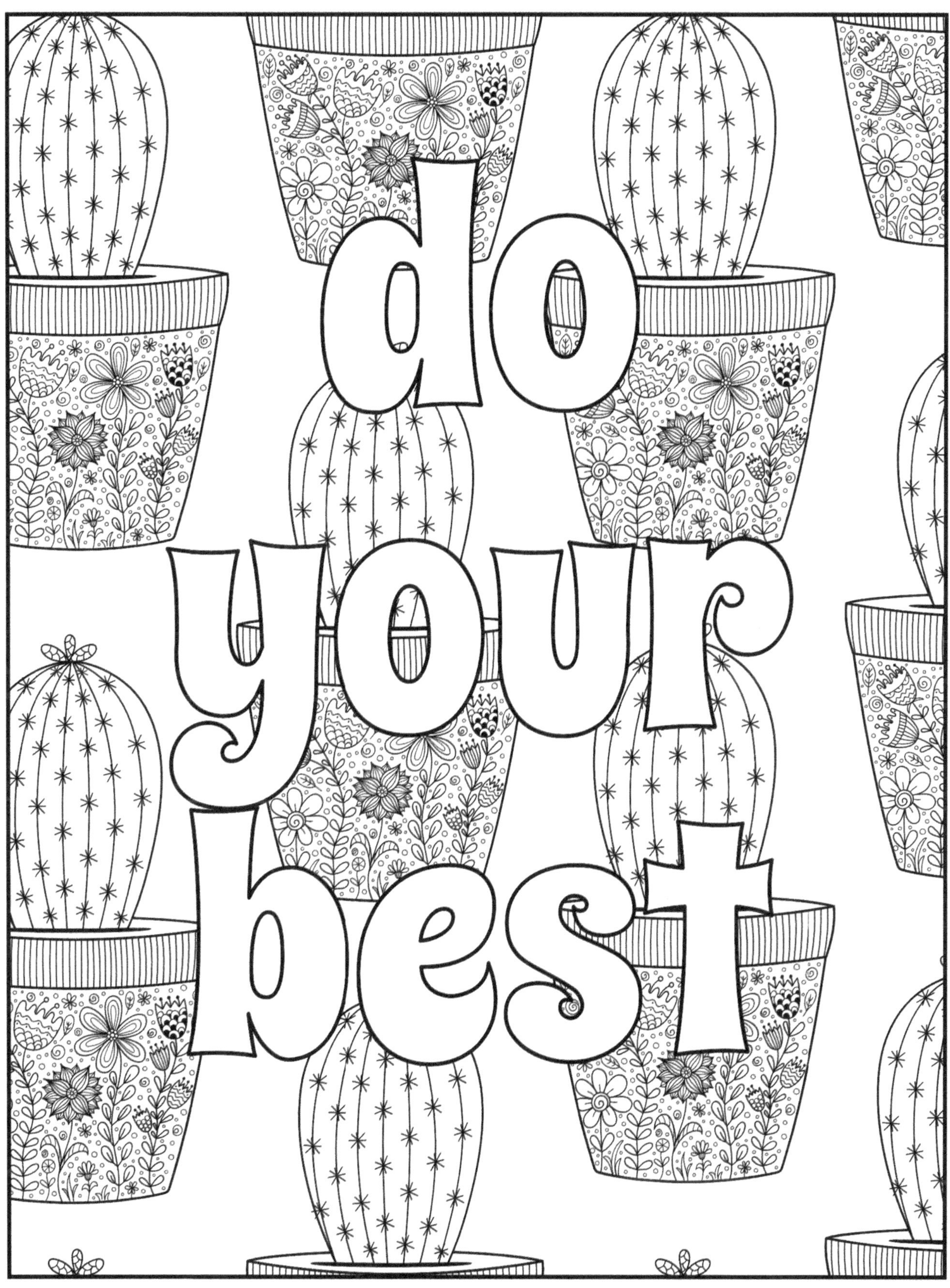

do your best

Blood Sugar Tracker

WEEK OF: _________________

Time	Before	After	Notes
Breakfast			
Lunch			
Dinner			
Bedtime			
Breakfast			
Lunch			
Dinner			
Bedtime			
Breakfast			
Lunch			
Dinner			
Bedtime			
Breakfast			
Lunch			
Dinner			
Bedtime			
Breakfast			
Lunch			
Dinner			
Bedtime			
Breakfast			
Lunch			
Dinner			
Bedtime			
Breakfast			
Lunch			
Dinner			
Bedtime			

Blood Sugar Tracker

WEEK OF: _________________

Time	Before	After	Notes
Breakfast			
Lunch			
Dinner			
Bedtime			
Breakfast			
Lunch			
Dinner			
Bedtime			
Breakfast			
Lunch			
Dinner			
Bedtime			
Breakfast			
Lunch			
Dinner			
Bedtime			
Breakfast			
Lunch			
Dinner			
Bedtime			
Breakfast			
Lunch			
Dinner			
Bedtime			
Breakfast			
Lunch			
Dinner			
Bedtime			

Blood Sugar Tracker

WEEK OF: ___________________

	Time	Before	After	Notes
Sunday	Breakfast Lunch Dinner Bedtime			
Monday	Breakfast Lunch Dinner Bedtime			
Tuesday	Breakfast Lunch Dinner Bedtime			
Wednesday	Breakfast Lunch Dinner Bedtime			
Thursday	Breakfast Lunch Dinner Bedtime			
Friday	Breakfast Lunch Dinner Bedtime			
Saturday	Breakfast Lunch Dinner Bedtime			

BLOOD SUGAR TRACKER

WEEK OF: _____________________

	Time	Before	After	Notes
Sunday	Breakfast			
	Lunch			
	Dinner			
	Bedtime			
Monday	Breakfast			
	Lunch			
	Dinner			
	Bedtime			
Tuesday	Breakfast			
	Lunch			
	Dinner			
	Bedtime			
Wednesday	Breakfast			
	Lunch			
	Dinner			
	Bedtime			
Thursday	Breakfast			
	Lunch			
	Dinner			
	Bedtime			
Friday	Breakfast			
	Lunch			
	Dinner			
	Bedtime			
Saturday	Breakfast			
	Lunch			
	Dinner			
	Bedtime			

NOTES:

Blood Sugar Tracker

WEEK OF: _______________

	Time	Before	After	Notes
	Breakfast			
	Lunch			
	Dinner			
	Bedtime			
	Breakfast			
	Lunch			
	Dinner			
	Bedtime			
	Breakfast			
	Lunch			
	Dinner			
	Bedtime			
	Breakfast			
	Lunch			
	Dinner			
	Bedtime			
	Breakfast			
	Lunch			
	Dinner			
	Bedtime			
	Breakfast			
	Lunch			
	Dinner			
	Bedtime			
	Breakfast			
	Lunch			
	Dinner			
	Bedtime			

Blood Sugar Tracker

	Time	Before	After	Notes
Sunday	Breakfast			
	Lunch			
	Dinner			
	Bedtime			
Monday	Breakfast			
	Lunch			
	Dinner			
	Bedtime			
Tuesday	Breakfast			
	Lunch			
	Dinner			
	Bedtime			
Wednesday	Breakfast			
	Lunch			
	Dinner			
	Bedtime			
Thursday	Breakfast			
	Lunch			
	Dinner			
	Bedtime			
Friday	Breakfast			
	Lunch			
	Dinner			
	Bedtime			
Saturday	Breakfast			
	Lunch			
	Dinner			
	Bedtime			

Blood Sugar Tracker

WEEK OF: _________________

	Time	Before	After	Notes
	Breakfast			
	Lunch			
	Dinner			
	Bedtime			
	Breakfast			
	Lunch			
	Dinner			
	Bedtime			
	Breakfast			
	Lunch			
	Dinner			
	Bedtime			
	Breakfast			
	Lunch			
	Dinner			
	Bedtime			
	Breakfast			
	Lunch			
	Dinner			
	Bedtime			
	Breakfast			
	Lunch			
	Dinner			
	Bedtime			
	Breakfast			
	Lunch			
	Dinner			
	Bedtime			

Blood Sugar Tracker

WEEK OF: _______________

<table>
<tr><th></th><th>Time</th><th>Before</th><th>After</th><th>Notes</th></tr>
<tr><td rowspan="4">Sunday</td><td>Breakfast</td><td></td><td></td><td></td></tr>
<tr><td>Lunch</td><td></td><td></td><td></td></tr>
<tr><td>Dinner</td><td></td><td></td><td></td></tr>
<tr><td>Bedtime</td><td></td><td></td><td></td></tr>
<tr><td rowspan="4">Monday</td><td>Breakfast</td><td></td><td></td><td></td></tr>
<tr><td>Lunch</td><td></td><td></td><td></td></tr>
<tr><td>Dinner</td><td></td><td></td><td></td></tr>
<tr><td>Bedtime</td><td></td><td></td><td></td></tr>
<tr><td rowspan="4">Tuesday</td><td>Breakfast</td><td></td><td></td><td></td></tr>
<tr><td>Lunch</td><td></td><td></td><td></td></tr>
<tr><td>Dinner</td><td></td><td></td><td></td></tr>
<tr><td>Bedtime</td><td></td><td></td><td></td></tr>
<tr><td rowspan="4">Wednesday</td><td>Breakfast</td><td></td><td></td><td></td></tr>
<tr><td>Lunch</td><td></td><td></td><td></td></tr>
<tr><td>Dinner</td><td></td><td></td><td></td></tr>
<tr><td>Bedtime</td><td></td><td></td><td></td></tr>
<tr><td rowspan="4">Thursday</td><td>Breakfast</td><td></td><td></td><td></td></tr>
<tr><td>Lunch</td><td></td><td></td><td></td></tr>
<tr><td>Dinner</td><td></td><td></td><td></td></tr>
<tr><td>Bedtime</td><td></td><td></td><td></td></tr>
<tr><td rowspan="4">Friday</td><td>Breakfast</td><td></td><td></td><td></td></tr>
<tr><td>Lunch</td><td></td><td></td><td></td></tr>
<tr><td>Dinner</td><td></td><td></td><td></td></tr>
<tr><td>Bedtime</td><td></td><td></td><td></td></tr>
<tr><td rowspan="4">Saturday</td><td>Breakfast</td><td></td><td></td><td></td></tr>
<tr><td>Lunch</td><td></td><td></td><td></td></tr>
<tr><td>Dinner</td><td></td><td></td><td></td></tr>
<tr><td>Bedtime</td><td></td><td></td><td></td></tr>
</table>

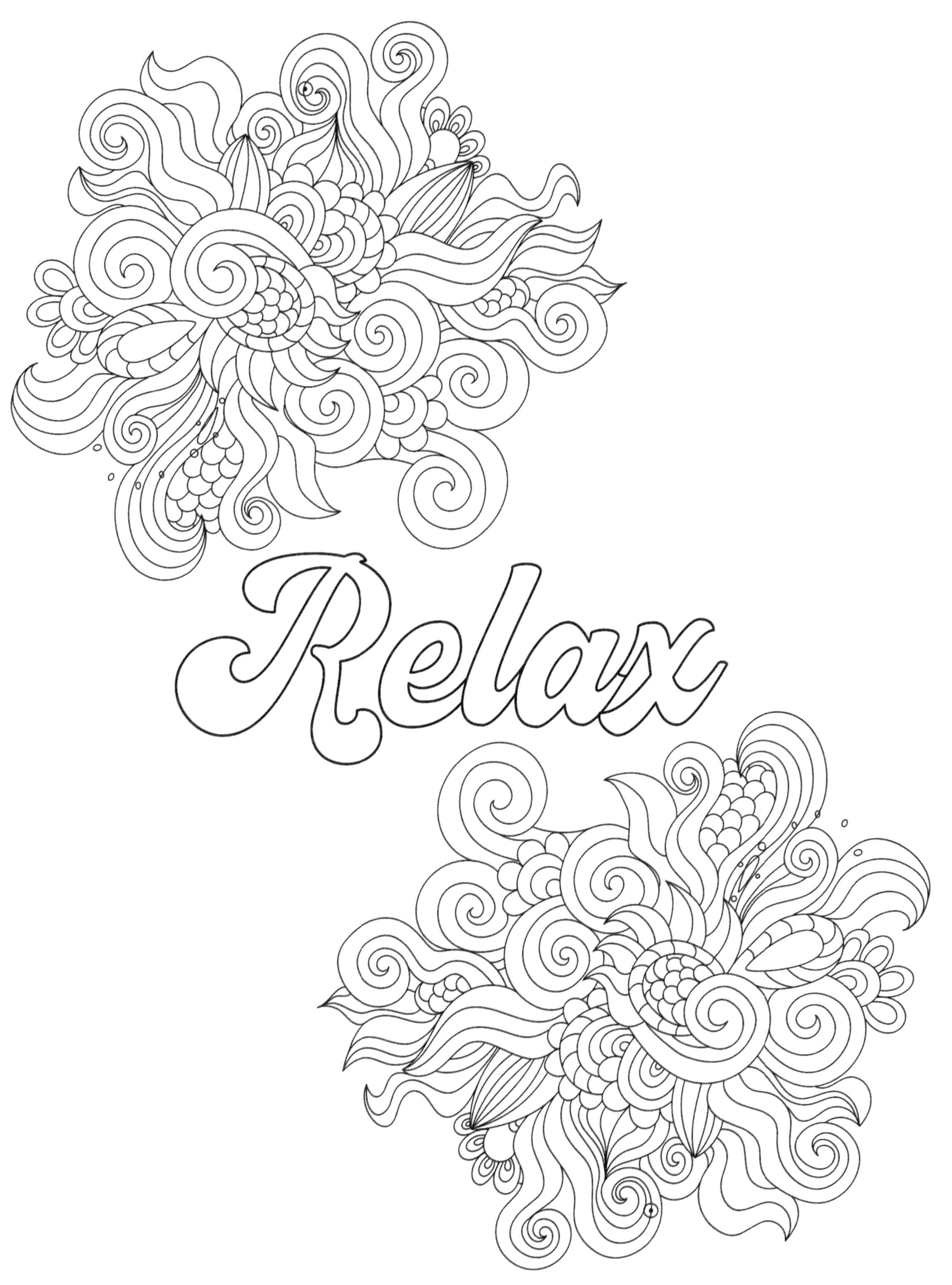
Relax

Blood Sugar Tracker

WEEK OF: ________________________

Time	Before	After	Notes
Breakfast			
Lunch			
Dinner			
Bedtime			
Breakfast			
Lunch			
Dinner			
Bedtime			
Breakfast			
Lunch			
Dinner			
Bedtime			
Breakfast			
Lunch			
Dinner			
Bedtime			
Breakfast			
Lunch			
Dinner			
Bedtime			
Breakfast			
Lunch			
Dinner			
Bedtime			
Breakfast			
Lunch			
Dinner			
Bedtime			

Blood Sugar Tracker

WEEK OF: _________________

	Time	Before	After	Notes
Sunday	Breakfast			
	Lunch			
	Dinner			
	Bedtime			
Monday	Breakfast			
	Lunch			
	Dinner			
	Bedtime			
Tuesday	Breakfast			
	Lunch			
	Dinner			
	Bedtime			
Wednesday	Breakfast			
	Lunch			
	Dinner			
	Bedtime			
Thursday	Breakfast			
	Lunch			
	Dinner			
	Bedtime			
Friday	Breakfast			
	Lunch			
	Dinner			
	Bedtime			
Saturday	Breakfast			
	Lunch			
	Dinner			
	Bedtime			

Blood Sugar Tracker

WEEK OF: _____________________

Day	Time	Before	After	Notes
Sunday	Breakfast			
	Lunch			
	Dinner			
	Bedtime			
Monday	Breakfast			
	Lunch			
	Dinner			
	Bedtime			
Tuesday	Breakfast			
	Lunch			
	Dinner			
	Bedtime			
Wednesday	Breakfast			
	Lunch			
	Dinner			
	Bedtime			
Thursday	Breakfast			
	Lunch			
	Dinner			
	Bedtime			
Friday	Breakfast			
	Lunch			
	Dinner			
	Bedtime			
Saturday	Breakfast			
	Lunch			
	Dinner			
	Bedtime			

Blood Sugar Tracker

WEEK OF: ________________________

	Time	Before	After	Notes
Sunday	Breakfast Lunch Dinner Bedtime			
Monday	Breakfast Lunch Dinner Bedtime			
Tuesday	Breakfast Lunch Dinner Bedtime			
Wednesday	Breakfast Lunch Dinner Bedtime			
Thursday	Breakfast Lunch Dinner Bedtime			
Friday	Breakfast Lunch Dinner Bedtime			
Saturday	Breakfast Lunch Dinner Bedtime			

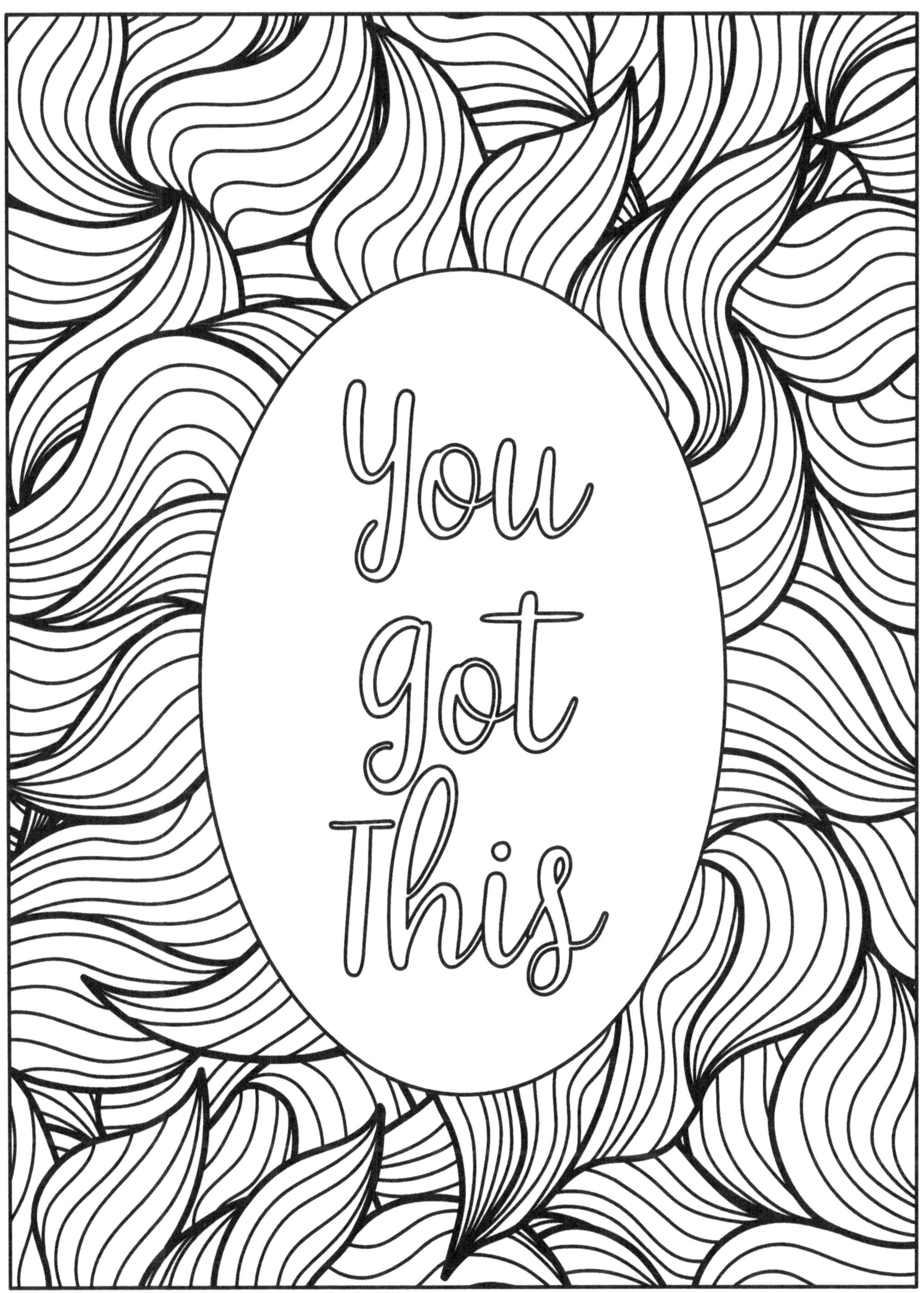
You
got
This

Blood Sugar Tracker

WEEK OF: _____________________

	Time	Before	After	Notes
	Breakfast			
	Lunch			
	Dinner			
	Bedtime			
	Breakfast			
	Lunch			
	Dinner			
	Bedtime			
	Breakfast			
	Lunch			
	Dinner			
	Bedtime			
	Breakfast			
	Lunch			
	Dinner			
	Bedtime			
	Breakfast			
	Lunch			
	Dinner			
	Bedtime			
	Breakfast			
	Lunch			
	Dinner			
	Bedtime			
	Breakfast			
	Lunch			
	Dinner			
	Bedtime			

Blood Sugar Tracker

WEEK OF: _______________________

	Time	Before	After	Notes
Sunday	Breakfast Lunch Dinner Bedtime			
Monday	Breakfast Lunch Dinner Bedtime			
Tuesday	Breakfast Lunch Dinner Bedtime			
Wednesday	Breakfast Lunch Dinner Bedtime			
Thursday	Breakfast Lunch Dinner Bedtime			
Friday	Breakfast Lunch Dinner Bedtime			
Saturday	Breakfast Lunch Dinner Bedtime			

Blood Sugar Tracker

WEEK OF: _______________

	Time	Before	After	Notes
	Breakfast			
	Lunch			
	Dinner			
	Bedtime			
	Breakfast			
	Lunch			
	Dinner			
	Bedtime			
	Breakfast			
	Lunch			
	Dinner			
	Bedtime			
	Breakfast			
	Lunch			
	Dinner			
	Bedtime			
	Breakfast			
	Lunch			
	Dinner			
	Bedtime			
	Breakfast			
	Lunch			
	Dinner			
	Bedtime			
	Breakfast			
	Lunch			
	Dinner			
	Bedtime			

Blood Sugar Tracker

WEEK OF: _________________

Day	Time	Before	After	Notes
Sunday	Breakfast			
	Lunch			
	Dinner			
	Bedtime			
Monday	Breakfast			
	Lunch			
	Dinner			
	Bedtime			
Tuesday	Breakfast			
	Lunch			
	Dinner			
	Bedtime			
Wednesday	Breakfast			
	Lunch			
	Dinner			
	Bedtime			
Thursday	Breakfast			
	Lunch			
	Dinner			
	Bedtime			
Friday	Breakfast			
	Lunch			
	Dinner			
	Bedtime			
Saturday	Breakfast			
	Lunch			
	Dinner			
	Bedtime			

NOTES:

www.ingramcontent.com/pod-product-compliance
Lightning Source LLC
Chambersburg PA
CBHW080522030726
47592CB00012B/3445